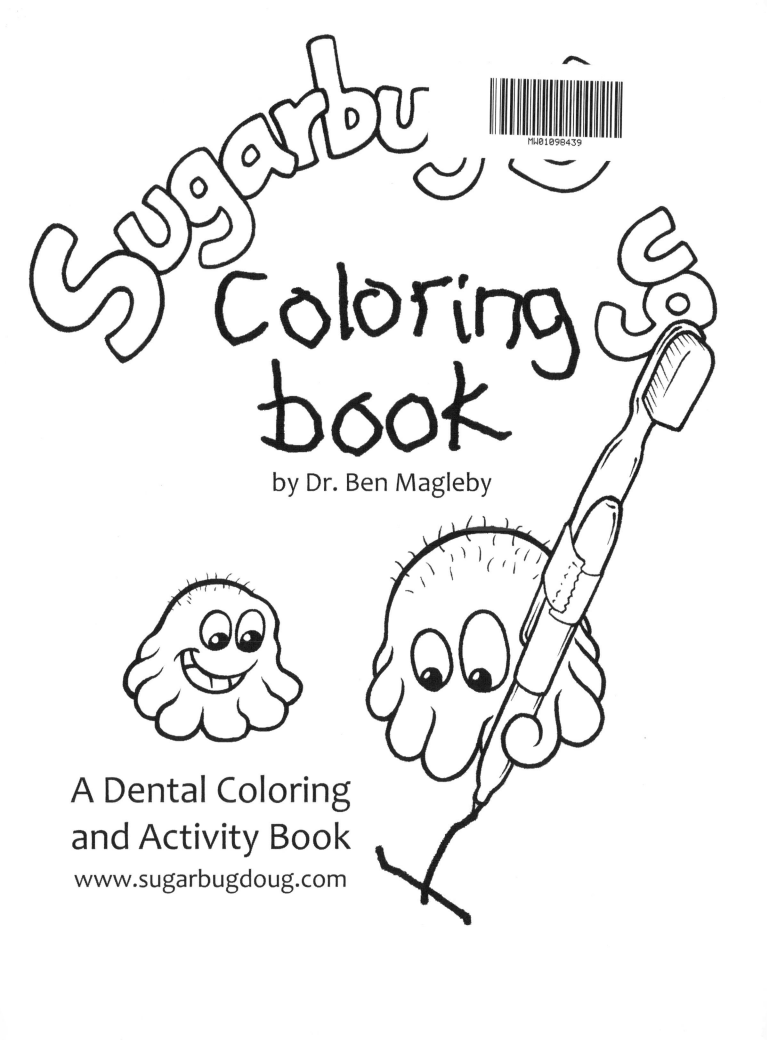

Sugarbu Coloring book

by Dr. Ben Magleby

A Dental Coloring
and Activity Book

www.sugarbugdoug.com

Illustrations were hand drawn and edited digitally.

Many of these pages can be found on the website, along with new additions.

www.sugarbugdoug.com

ISBN-13: 978-1535241984
ISBN-10: 1535241985

Printed by CreateSpace, an Amazon.com Company
Copyright 2016 Benjamin Magleby, D.D.S.

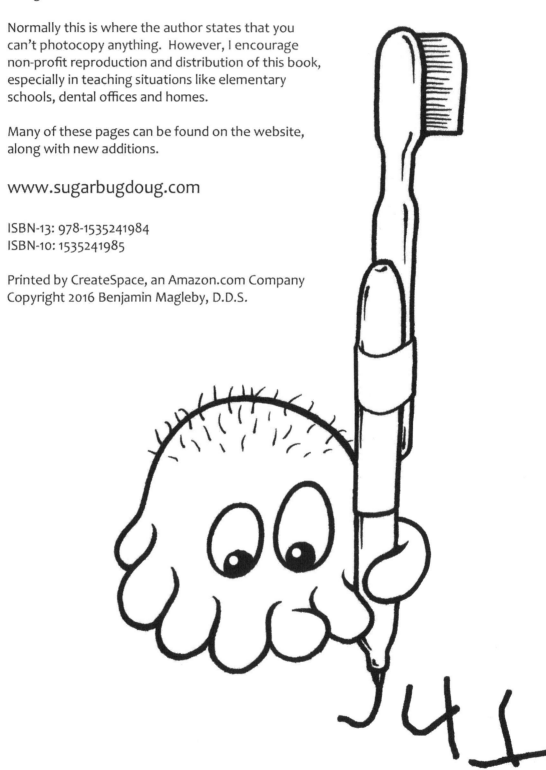

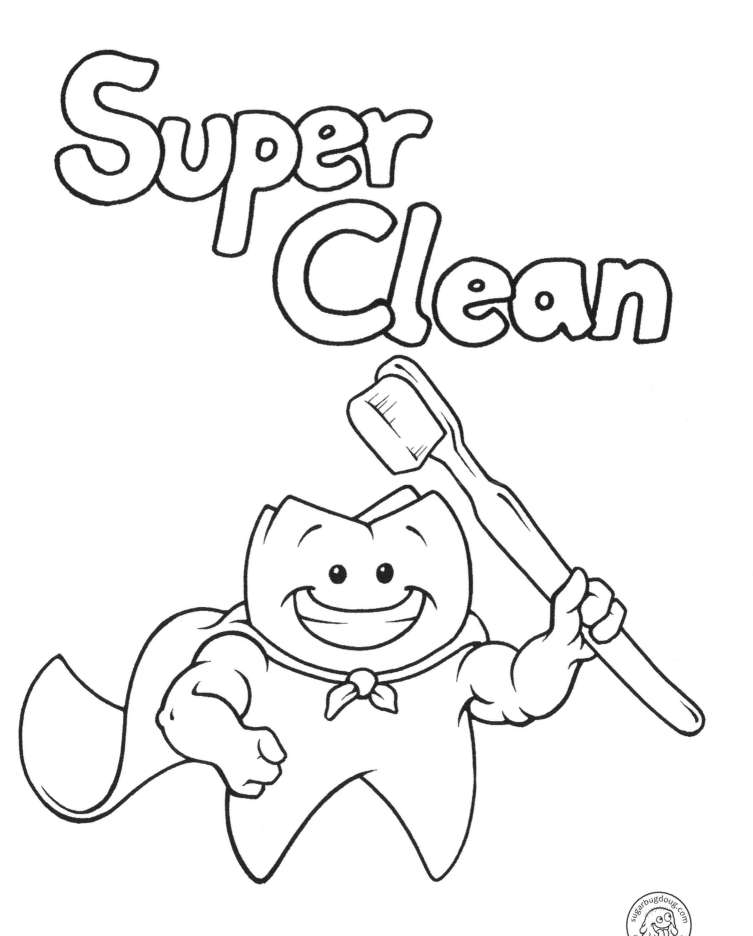

Cavity Fighter

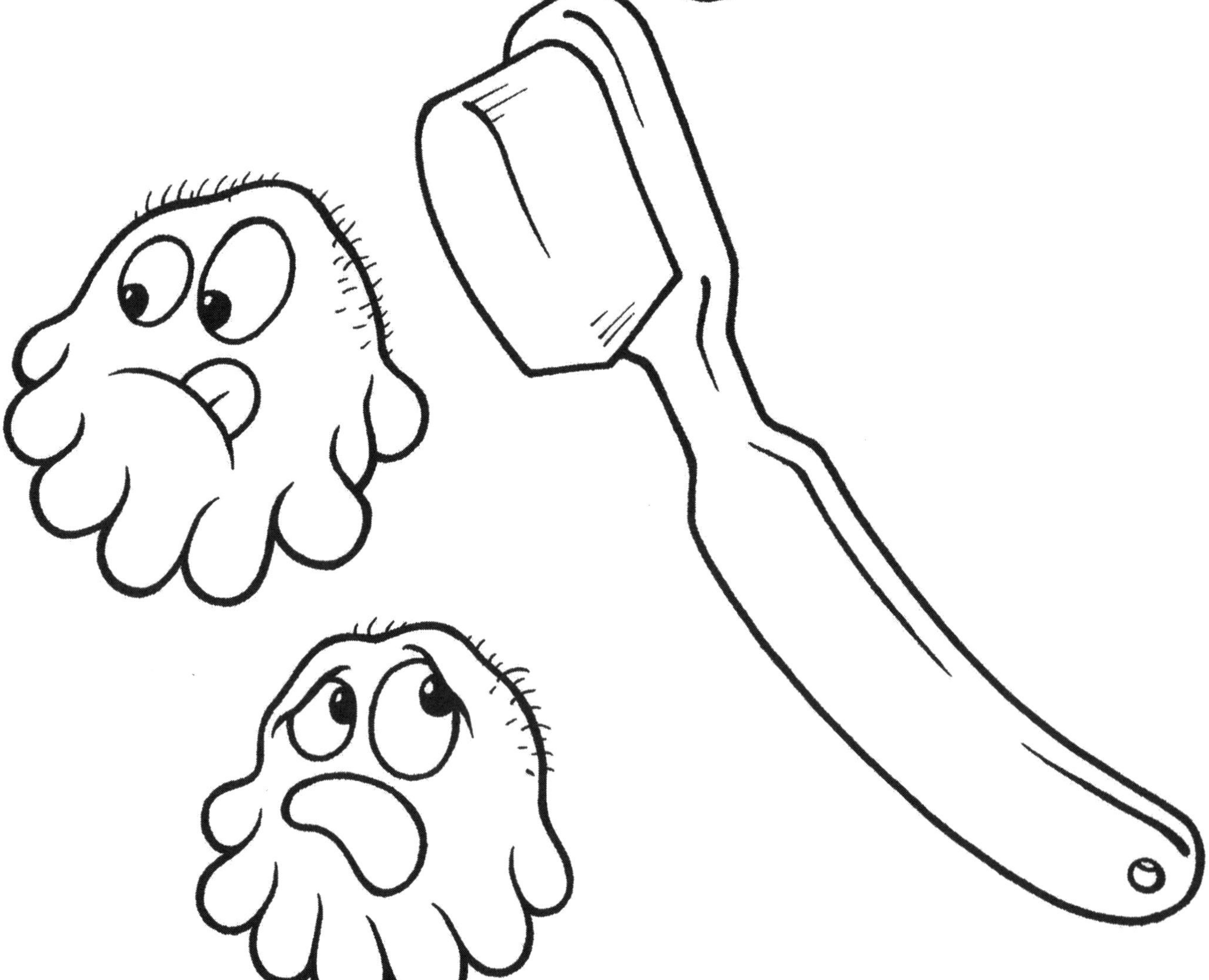

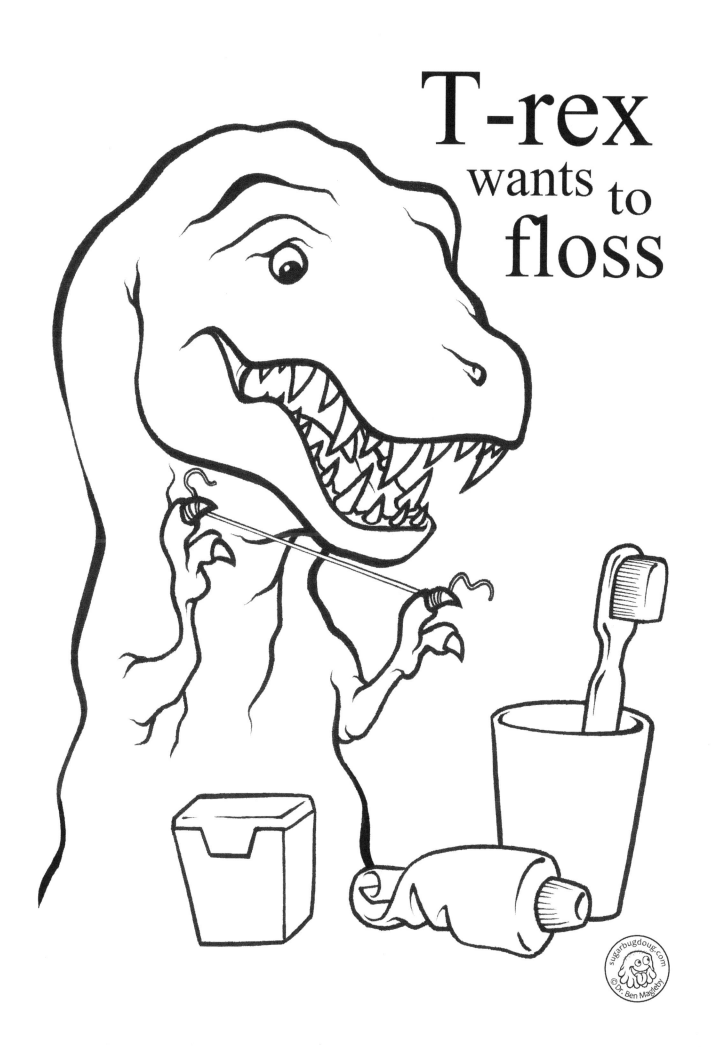

Every Toothsaurus

knows how important it is to

brush back teeth!

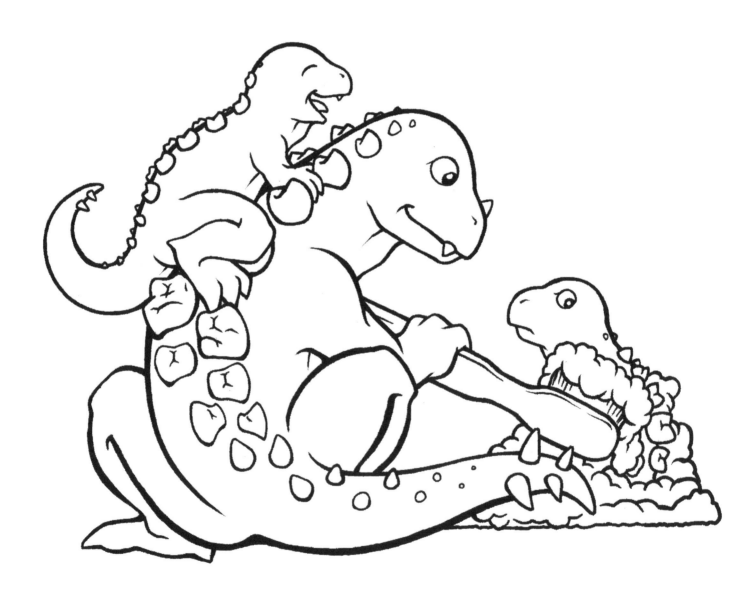

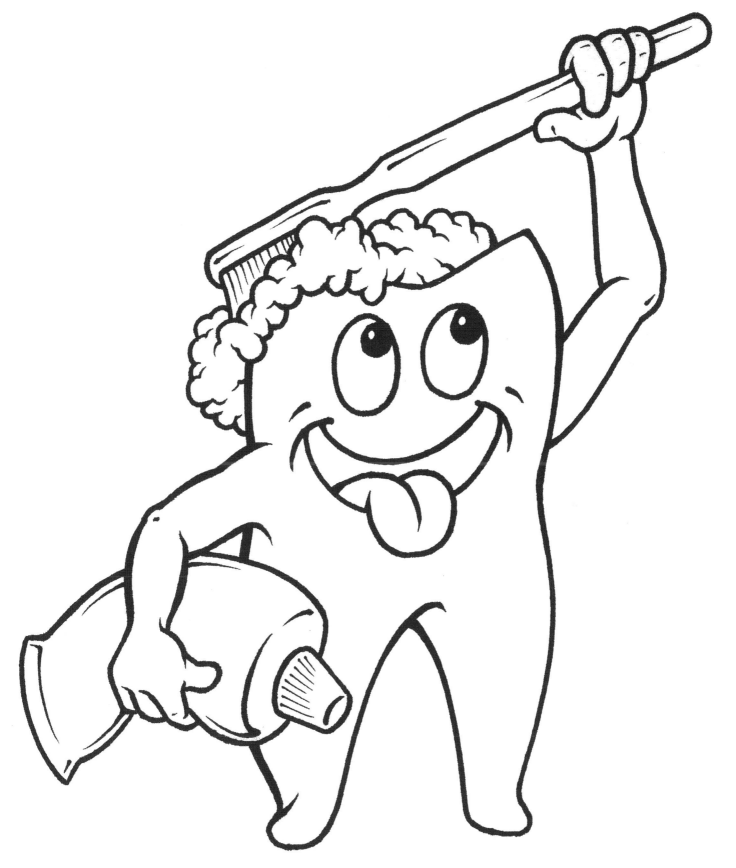

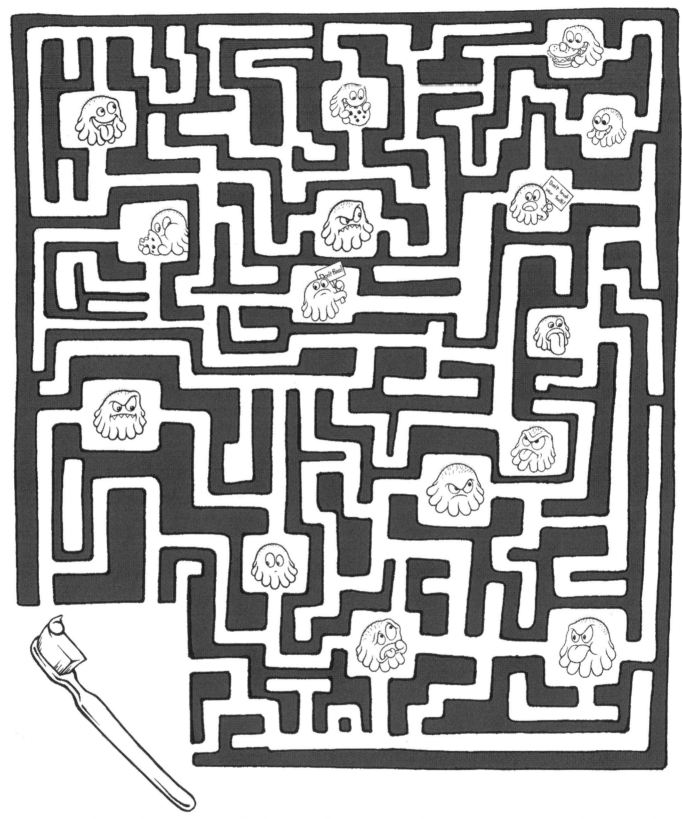

Help the toothbrush get all the sugarbugs!

Brushing your Teeth

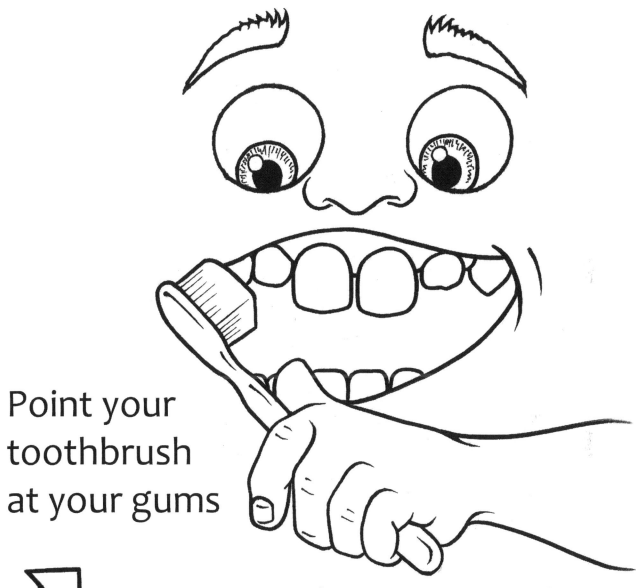

Point your
toothbrush
at your gums

 Point up at the upper teeth

 Point down at the lower teeth

 Brush in small circles

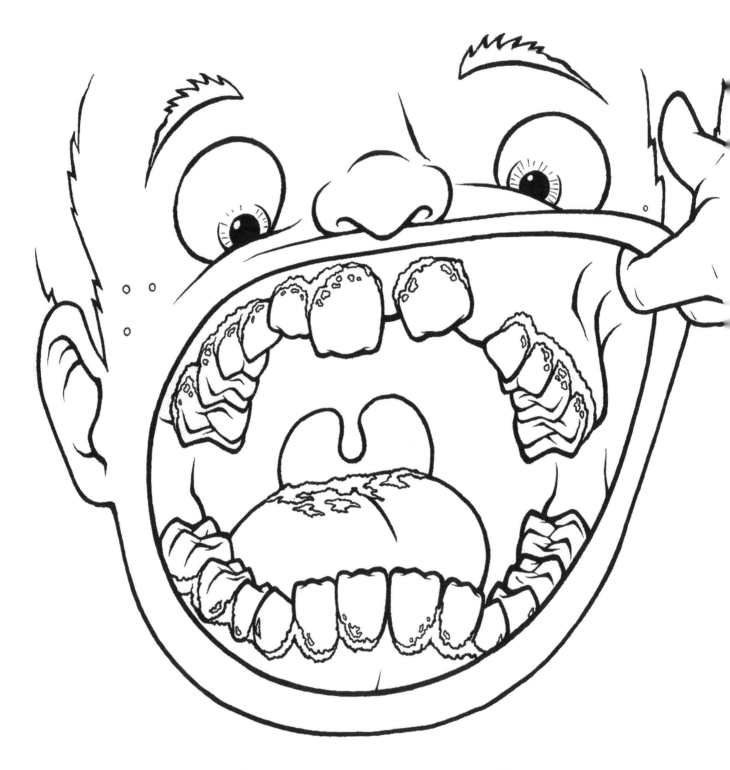

Plaque mouth

Toothbrush Pledge

I pledge allegiance to the brush,
to clean my teeth each day,
so I won't worry about cavities
when I go out to play.

I'll brush them every morning,
and each and every night.
I'll be sure to floss them in-between,
before turning out my light.

Eating good and healthy food,
like fruits and veggies too,
helps to keep my teeth real clean,
each and every time I chew.

I'll keep on brushing every day,
to show my teeth I care,
that way when I'm older,
my teeth will still be there.

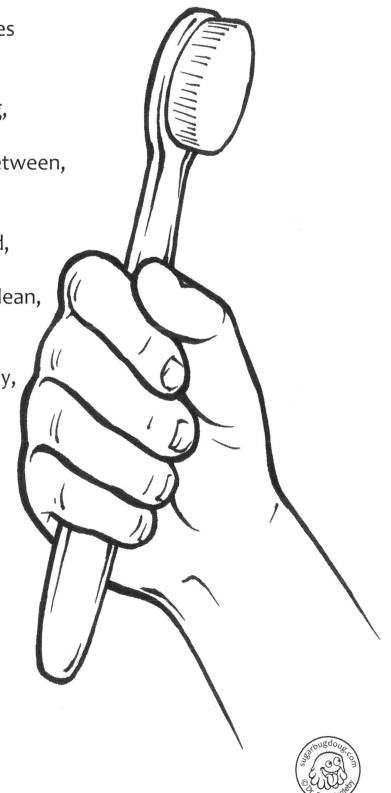

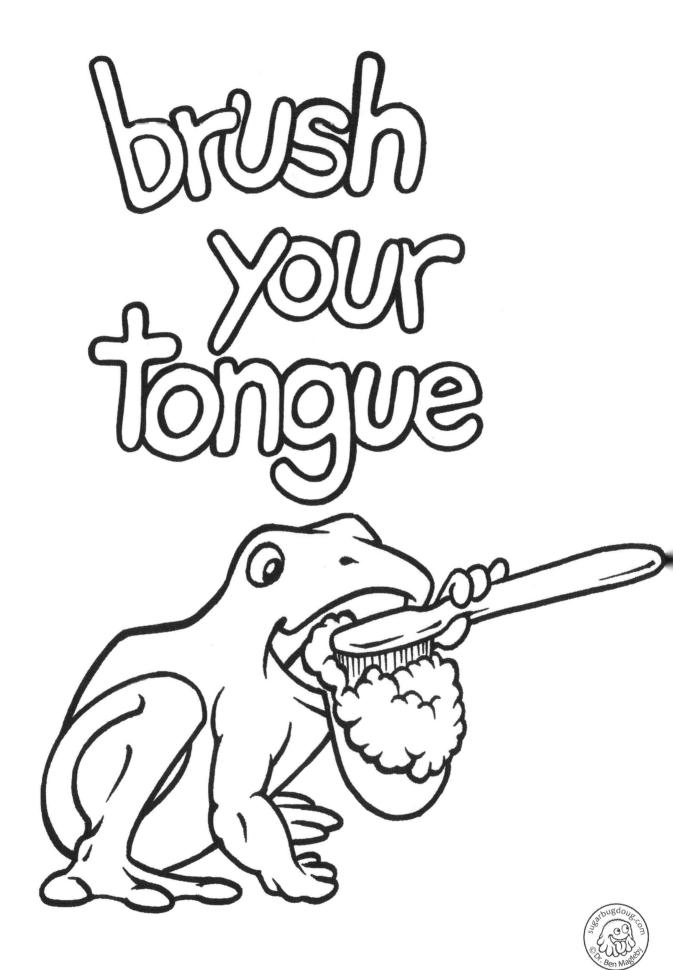

Clean Teeth Chart

Cross out a sugarbug every day that you
brush your teeth morning and night
and floss at least once

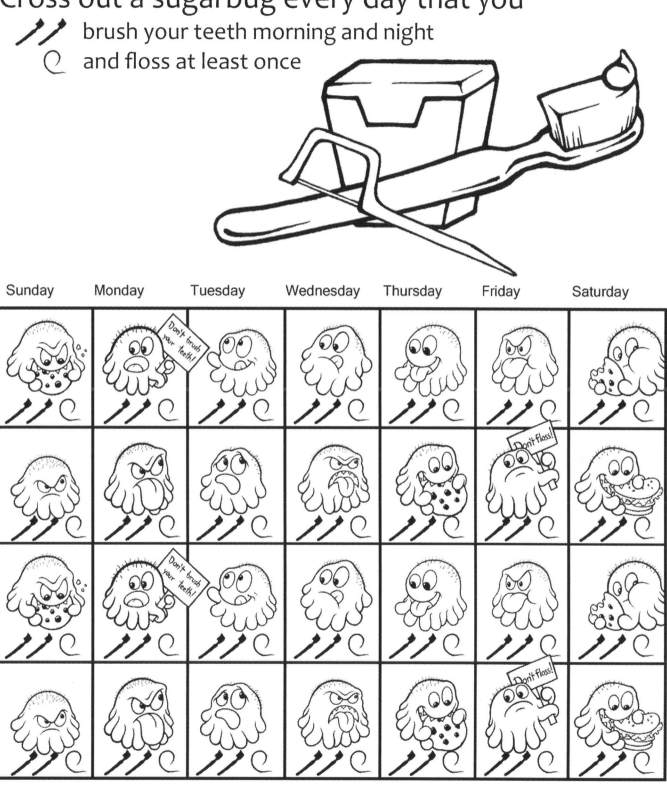

Sunday	Monday	Tuesday	Wednesday	Thursday	Friday	Saturday

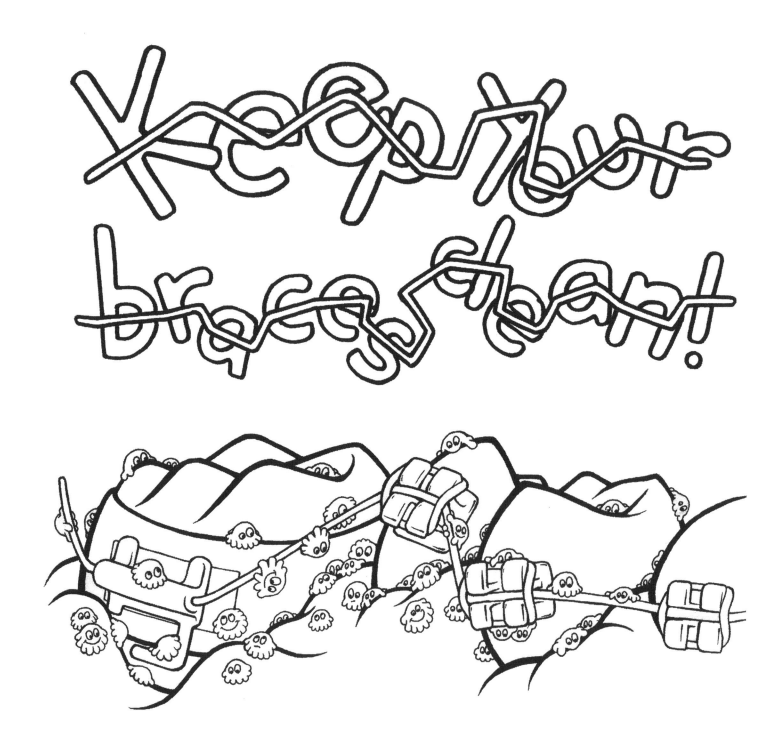

Flossing your Teeth

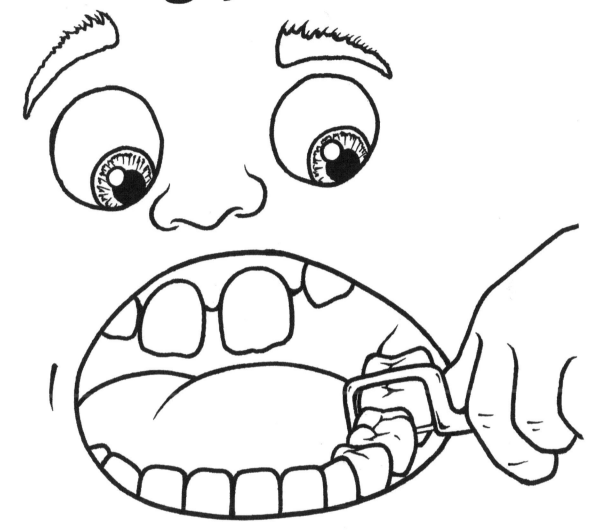

○ Floss all your teeth,
especially all teeth that touch

○ Most importantly,
floss all grown up teeth

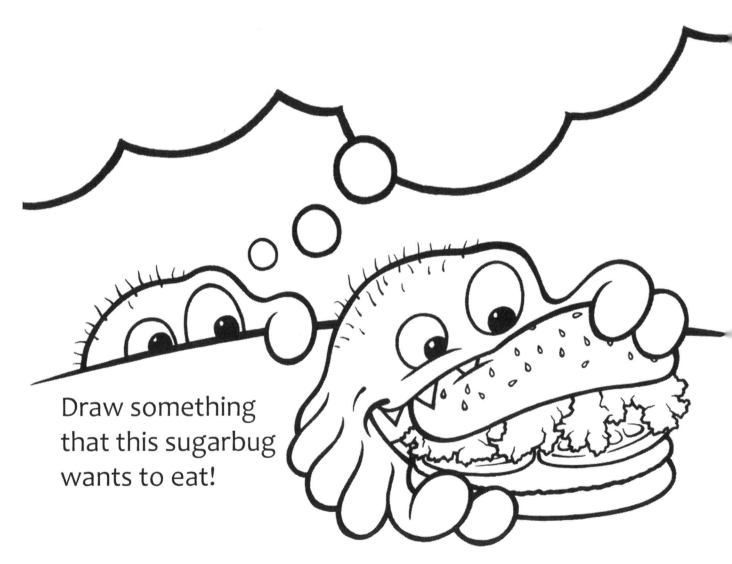

Draw something that this sugarbug wants to eat!

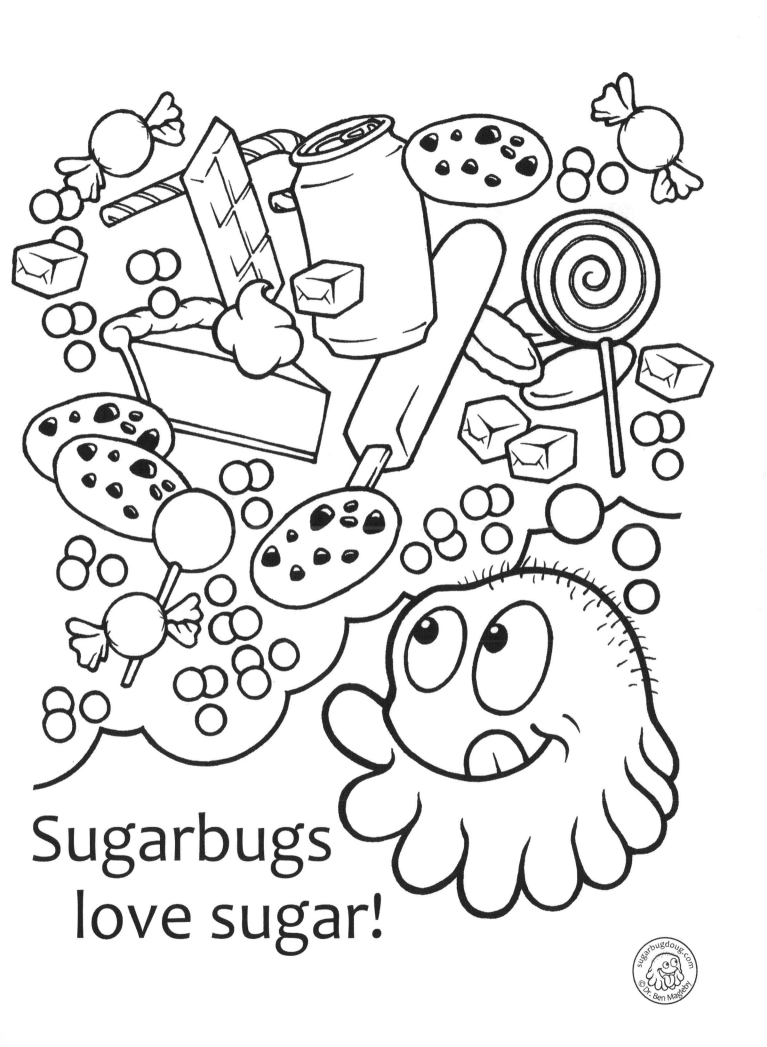

Sugarbugs
love sugar!

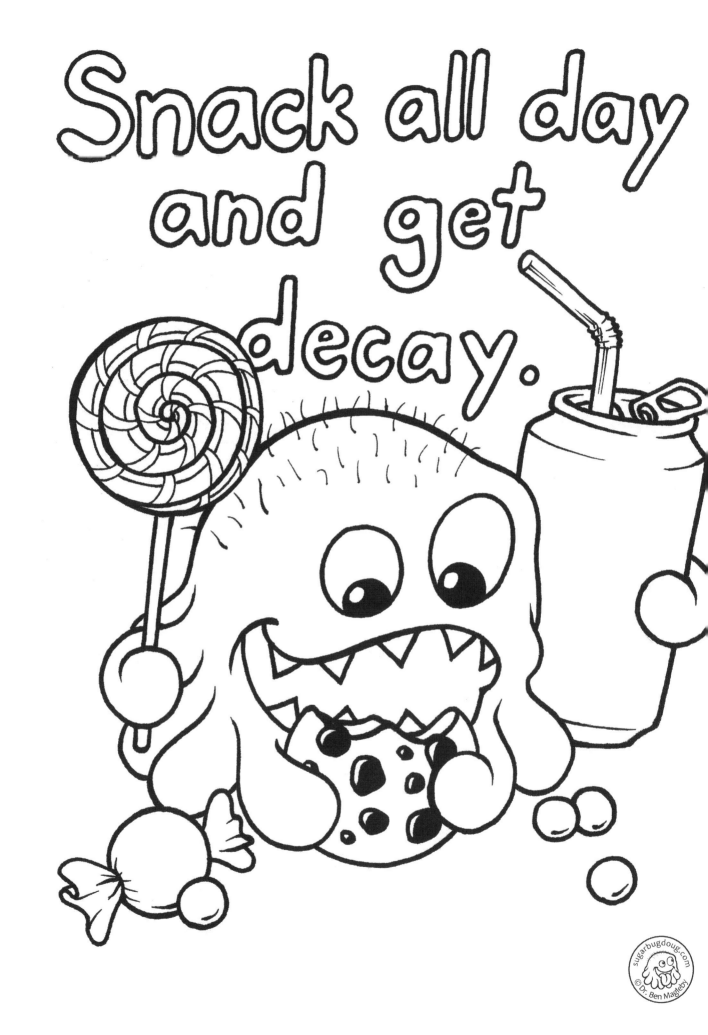

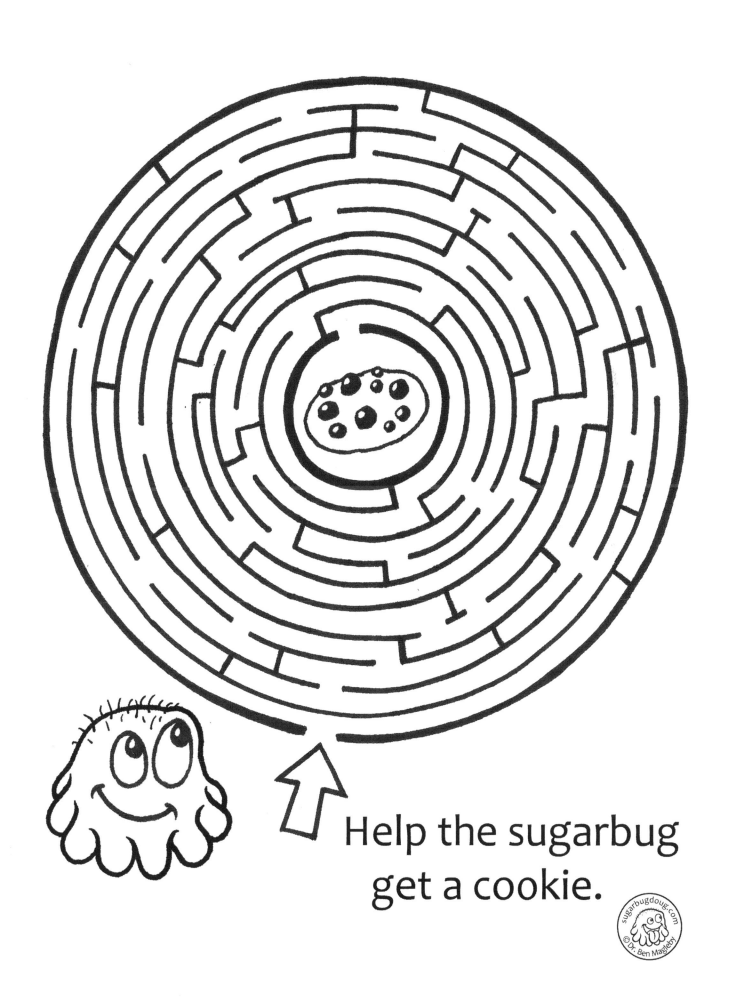

Help the sugarbug
get a cookie.

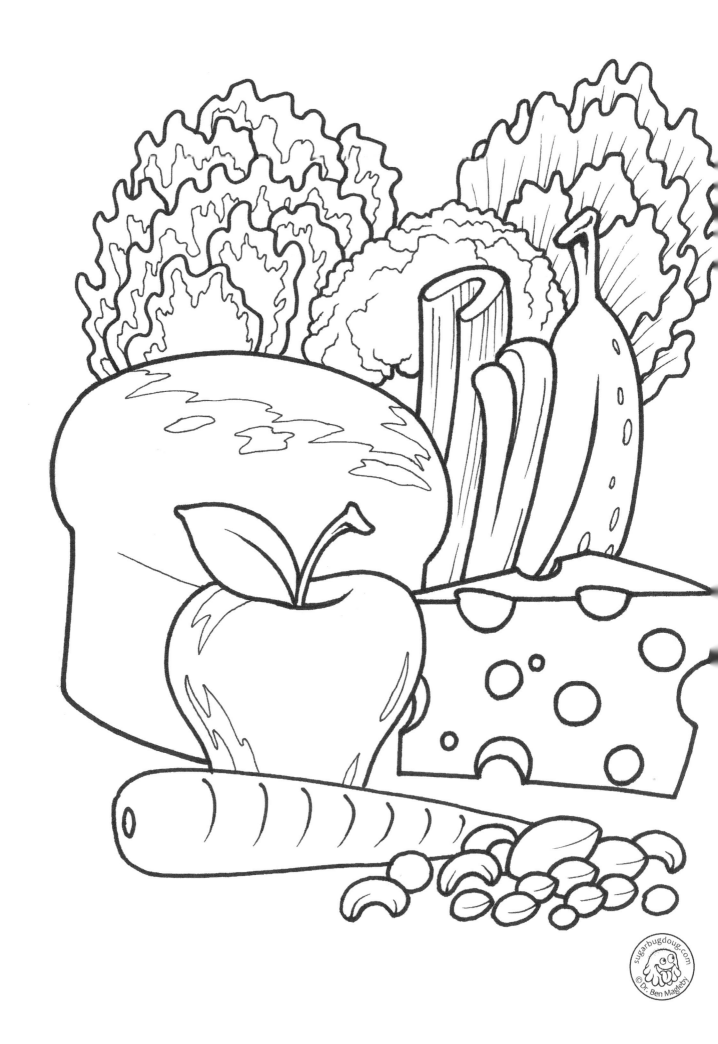

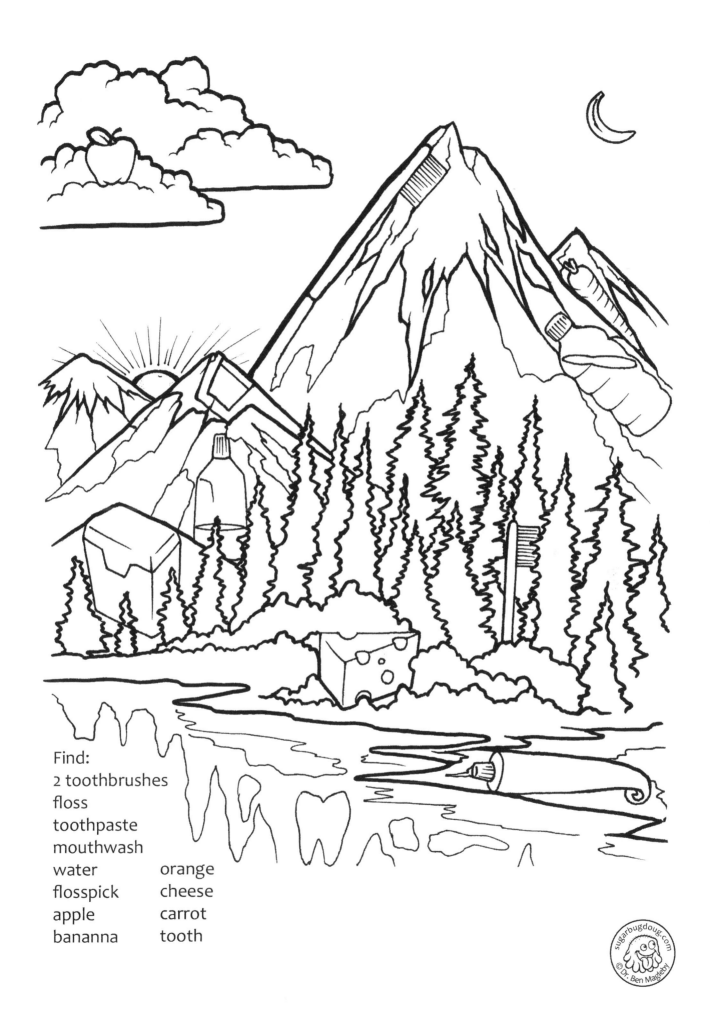

Find:
2 toothbrushes
floss
toothpaste
mouthwash
water   orange
flosspick   cheese
apple   carrot
bananna   tooth

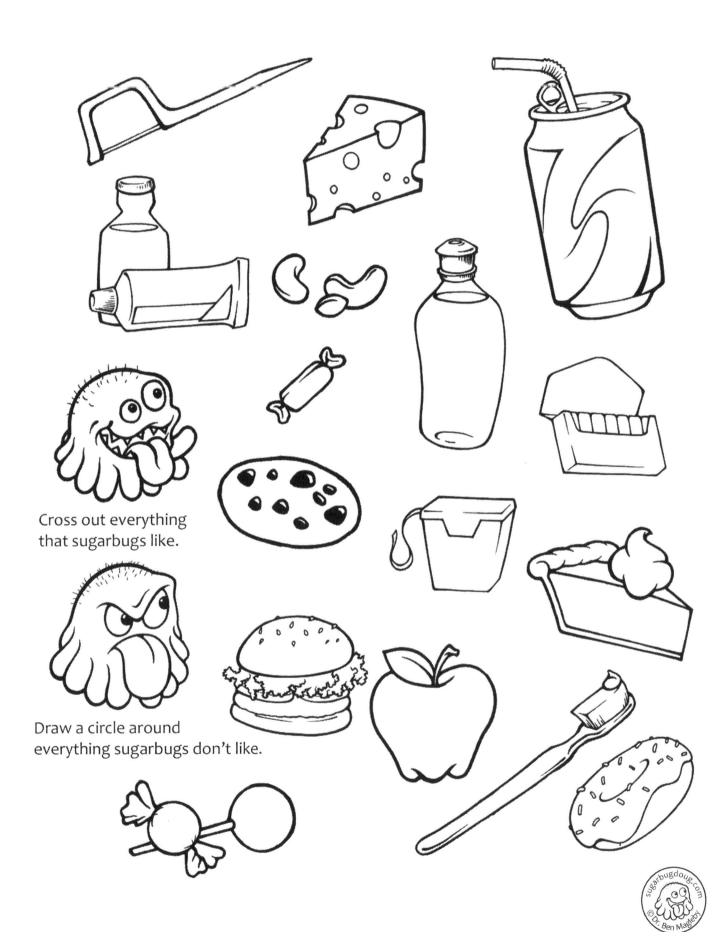

Cross out everything
that sugarbugs like.

Draw a circle around
everything sugarbugs don't like.

sugarbugdoug.com
© Dr. Ben Magleby

Sugarbugs can move from tooth to tooth and cause more cavities!

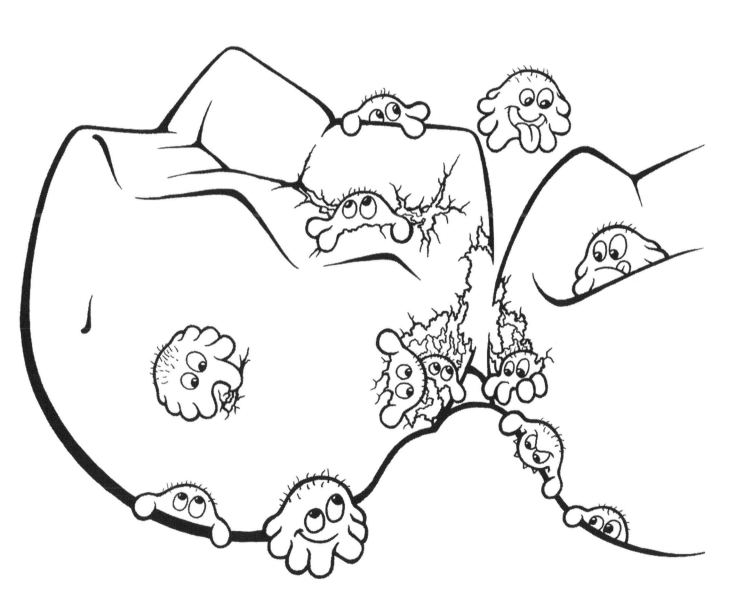

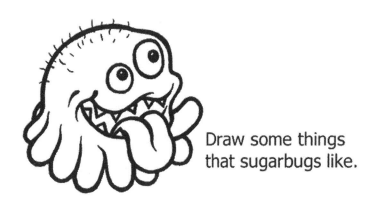

Draw some things
that sugarbugs like.

Draw some things that
sugarbugs don't like.

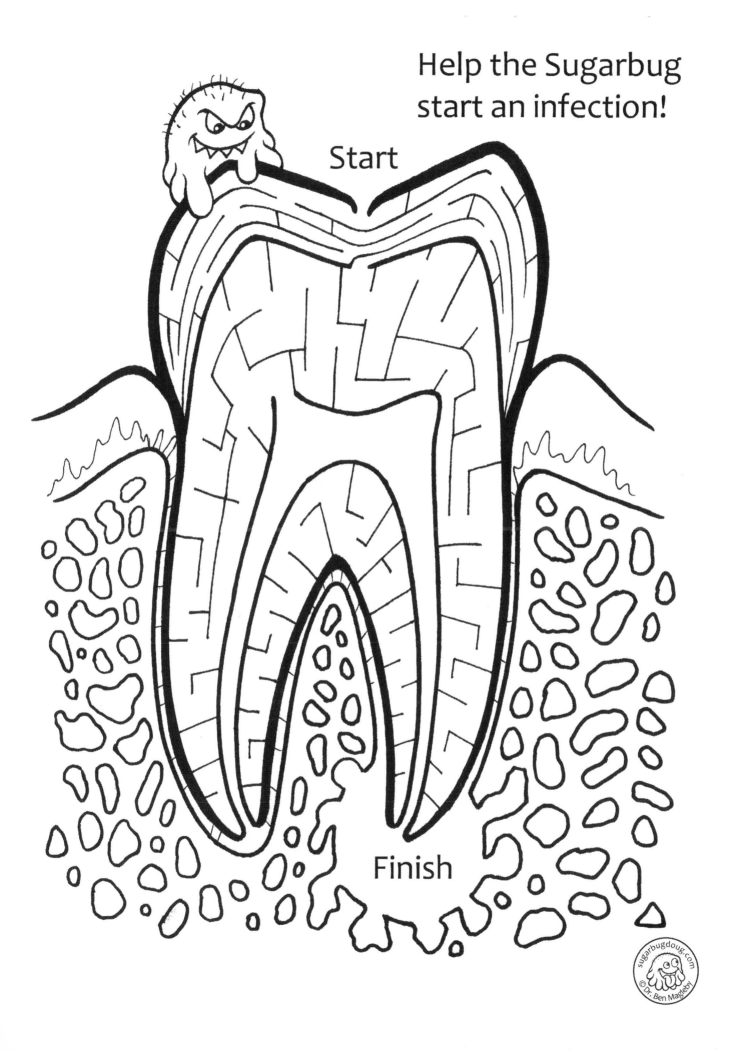

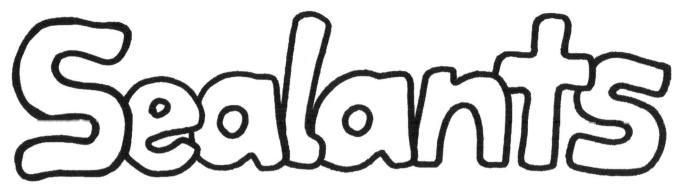

Sealants

Sealants protect teeth by filling in hard to clean grooves

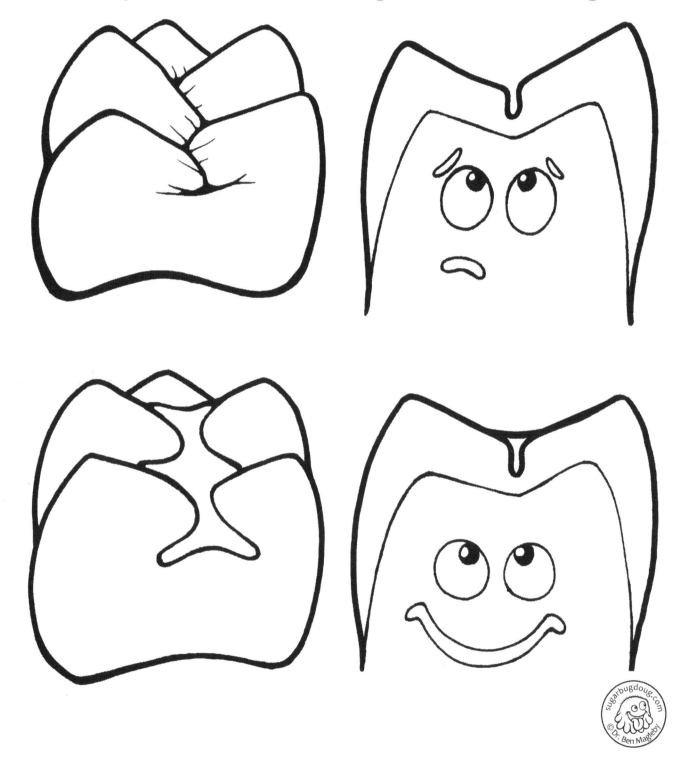

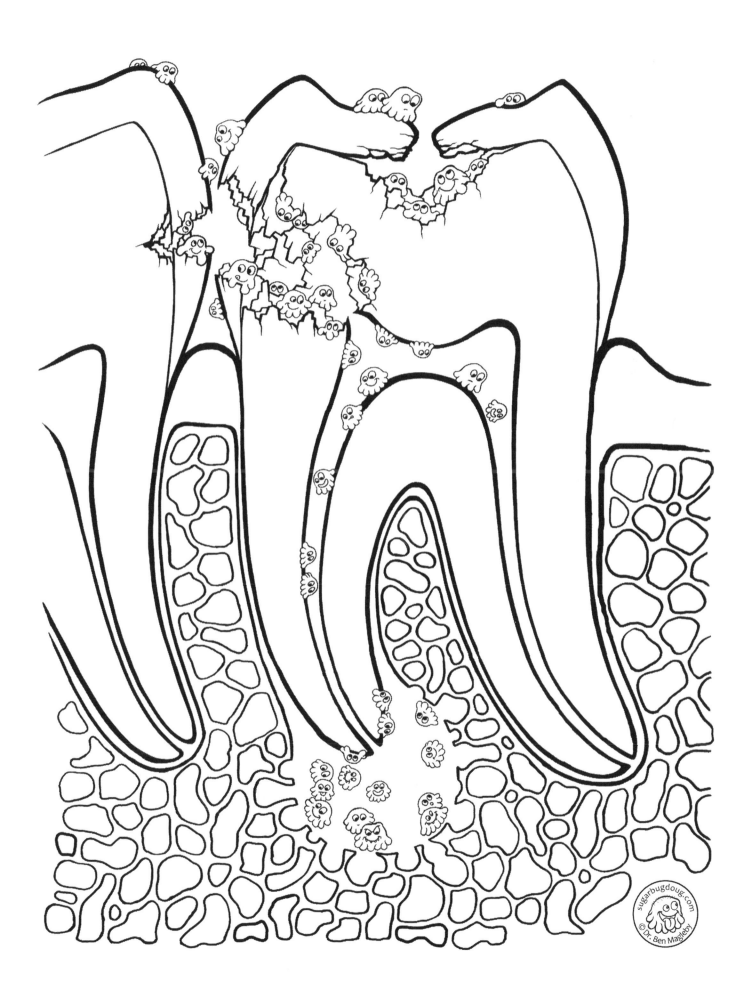

Find four matching pairs

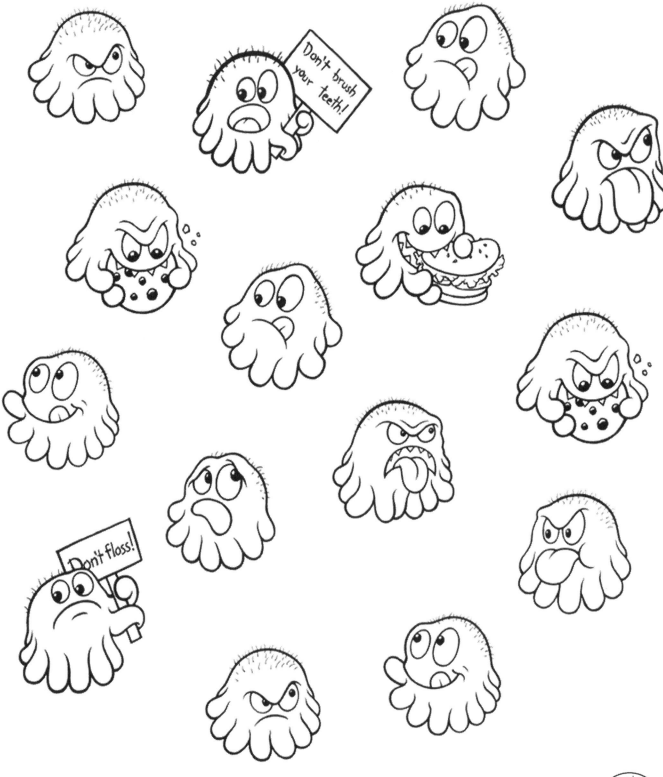

S	T	W	A	S	H	H	A	N	D	S	H
N	P	D	G	D	X	R	V	B	J	O	G
A	L	E	C	W	A	T	E	R	Z	D	H
C	A	N	D	Y	J	D	G	Z	C	A	E
K	Q	T	E	E	T	H	E	D	O	P	A
A	U	I	F	R	U	I	T	O	L	O	L
L	E	S	L	D	Z	O	A	B	A	P	T
L	Z	T	O	O	T	H	B	R	U	S	H
D	B	D	S	D	B	X	L	B	G	Z	Y
A	Z	O	S	M	I	L	E	O	H	R	S
Y	C	O	O	K	I	E	S	D	B	O	D
A	N	D	G	E	T	D	E	C	A	Y	O

Candy
Cookies
Dentist
Fruit
Healthy
Jog
Laugh
Plaque
Smile
Snack all day and
    get decay
Sodapop
Teeth
Toothbrush
Vegetables
Wash hands
Water

WORD SEARCH

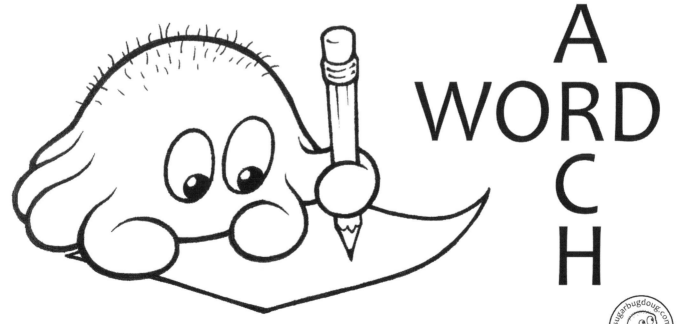

sugarbugdoug.com
© Dr. Ben Magleby

Dot-to-Dot

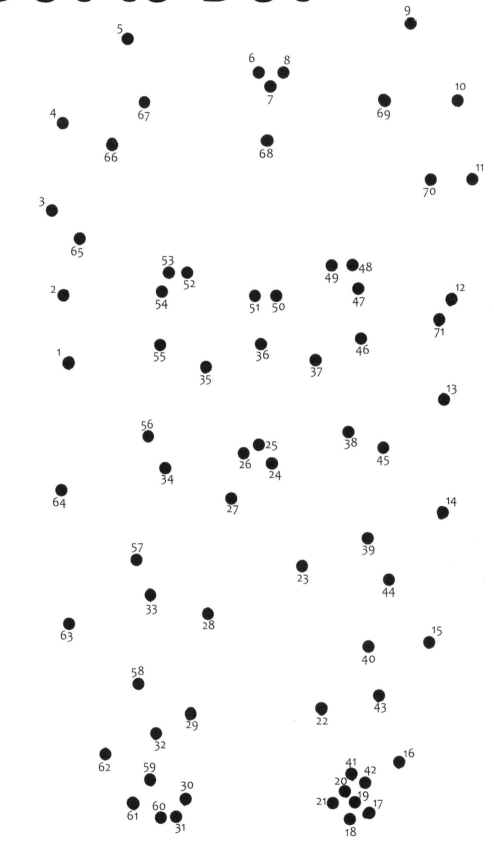

Find the one that's different

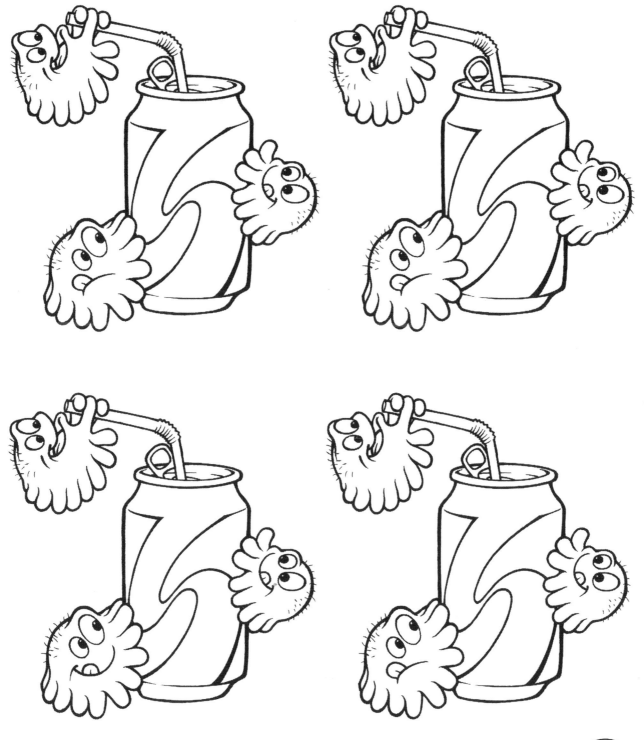

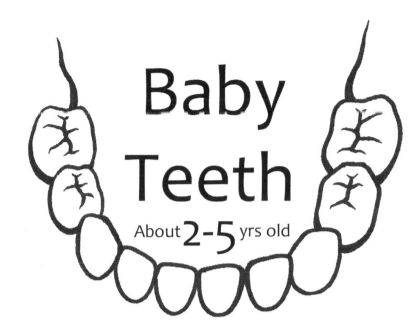

Baby Teeth
About 2-5 yrs old

Starting to get Grown up Teeth
About 7-10 yrs old

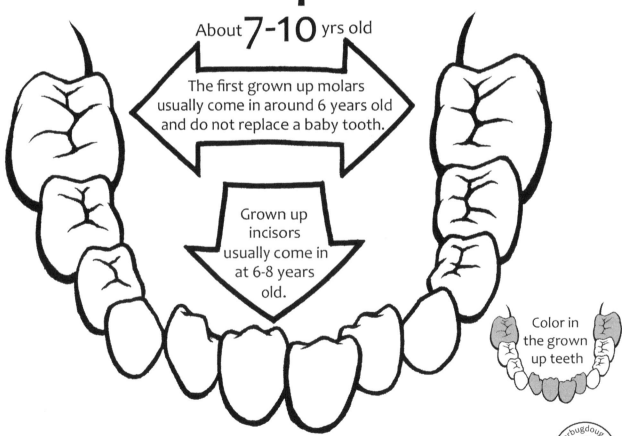

The first grown up molars usually come in around 6 years old and do not replace a baby tooth.

Grown up incisors usually come in at 6-8 years old.

Color in the grown up teeth

sugarbugdoug.com
©Dr. Ben Magleby

Losing Teeth

My first tooth was loose today,
I found when I woke up,
it wiggled back and forth
and fell into a cup.

My tooth space feels a little strange,
a hole that's fun and new.
I can put a straw in there
and use it through and through.

My grown up tooth came in,
as a little time went by,
if I keep it nice and clean,
it will be there 'til I die.

Teeth fall out and teeth come in,
before it's said and done.
It's all part of growing up,
and growing up is fun!

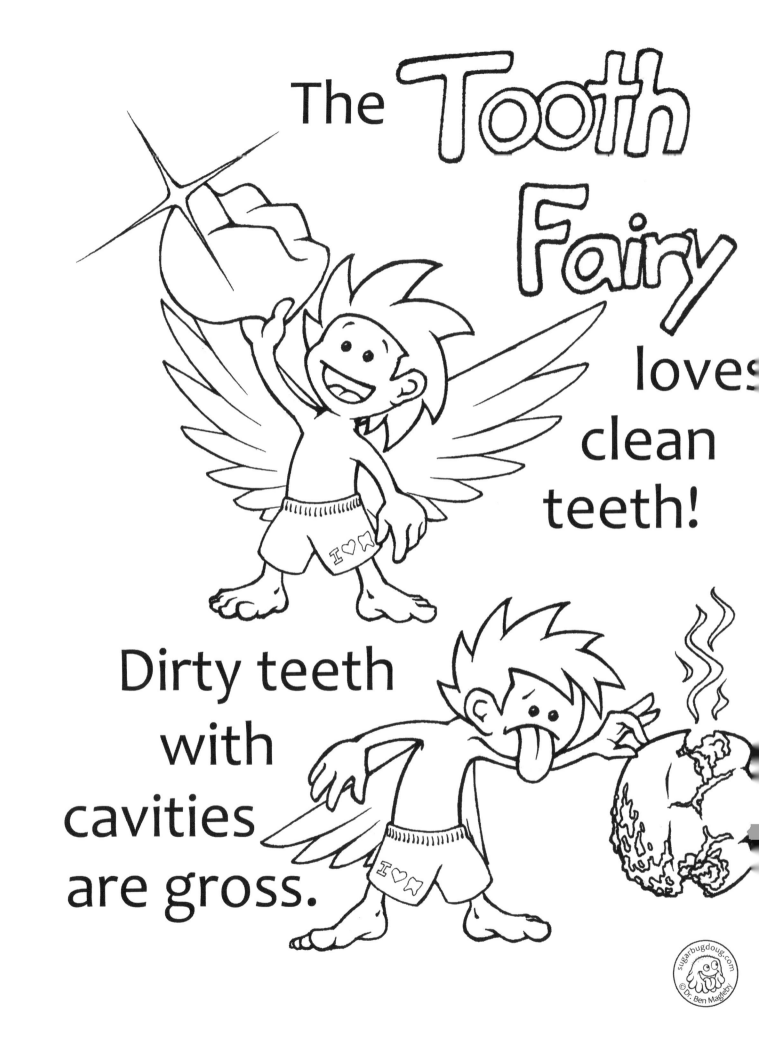

The Tooth Fairy loves clean teeth!

Dirty teeth with cavities are gross.

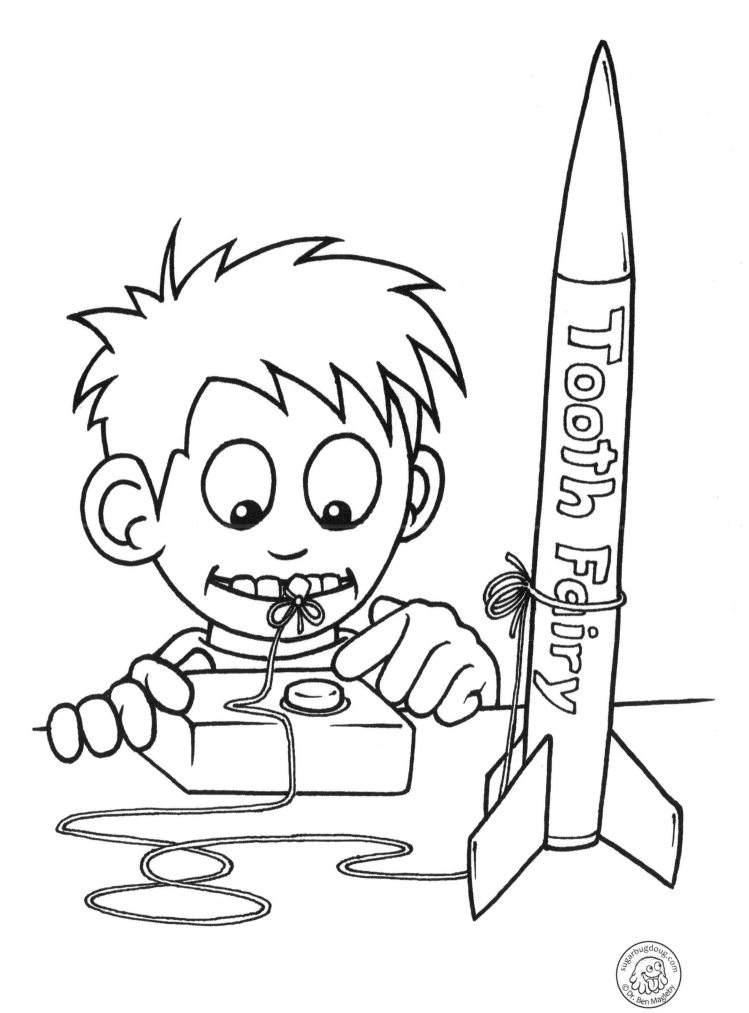

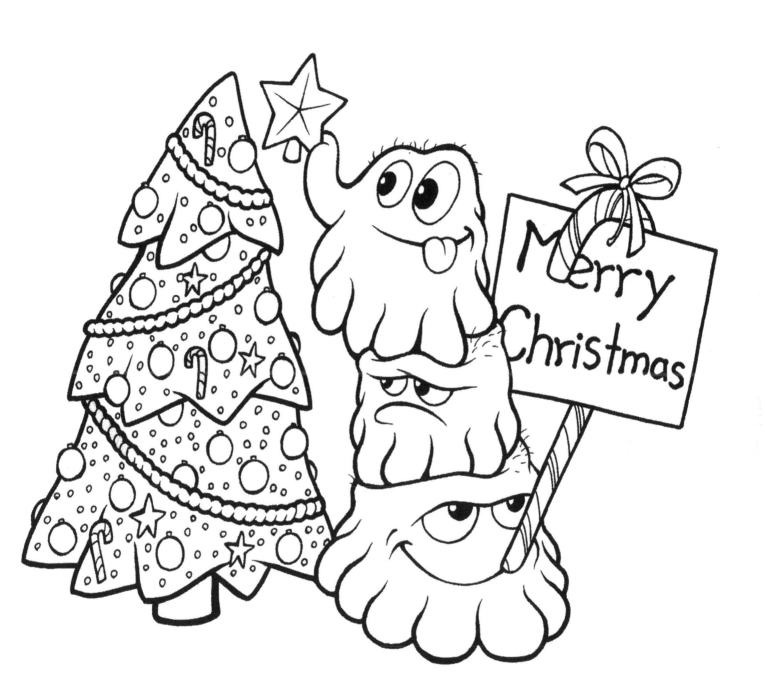

Happy 4th of July!

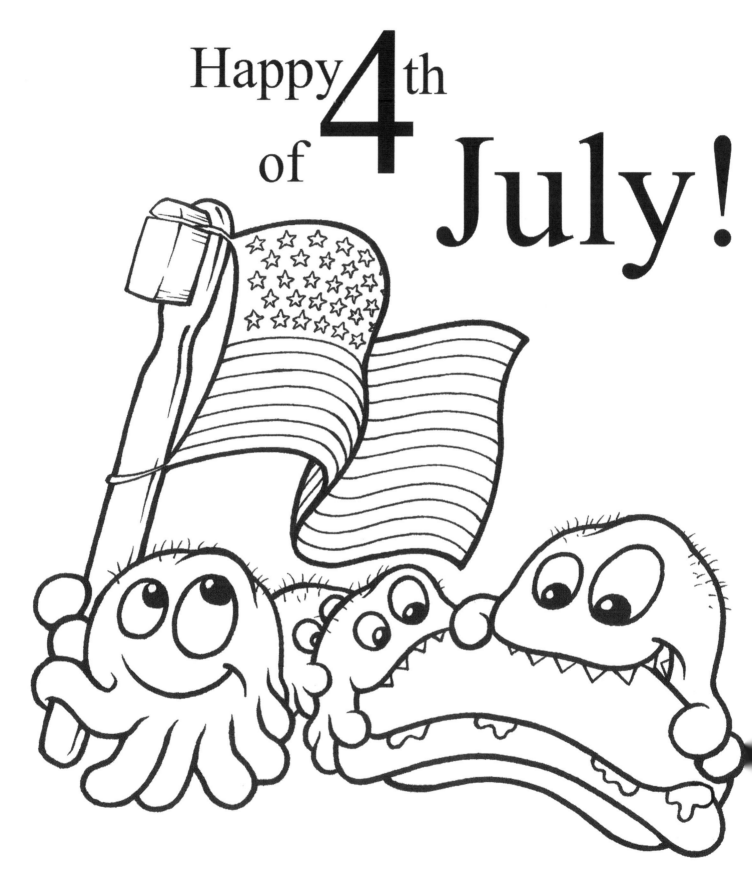

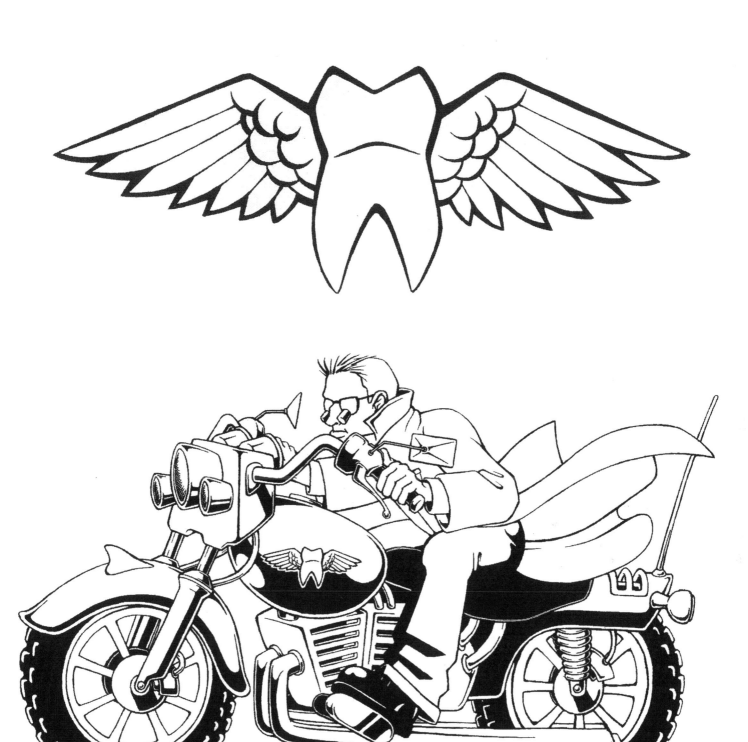

USE THE FLOSS, LUKE.

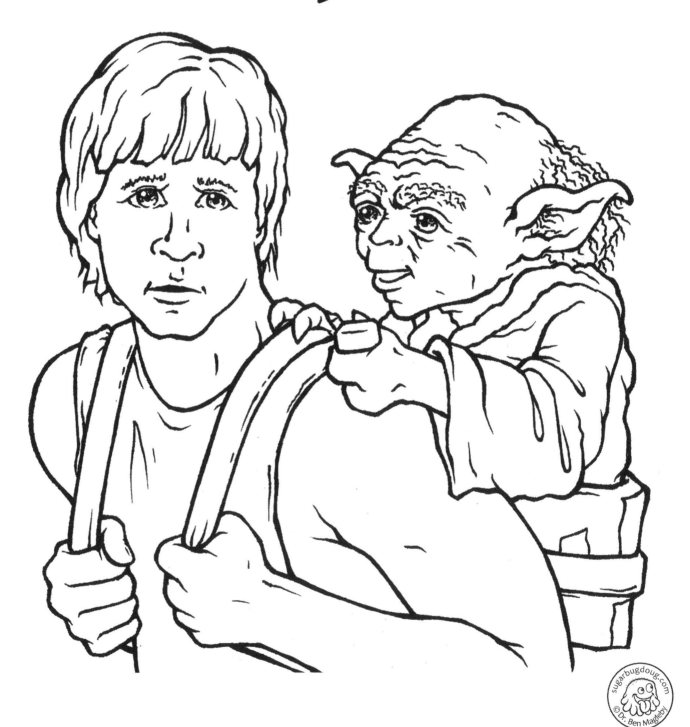

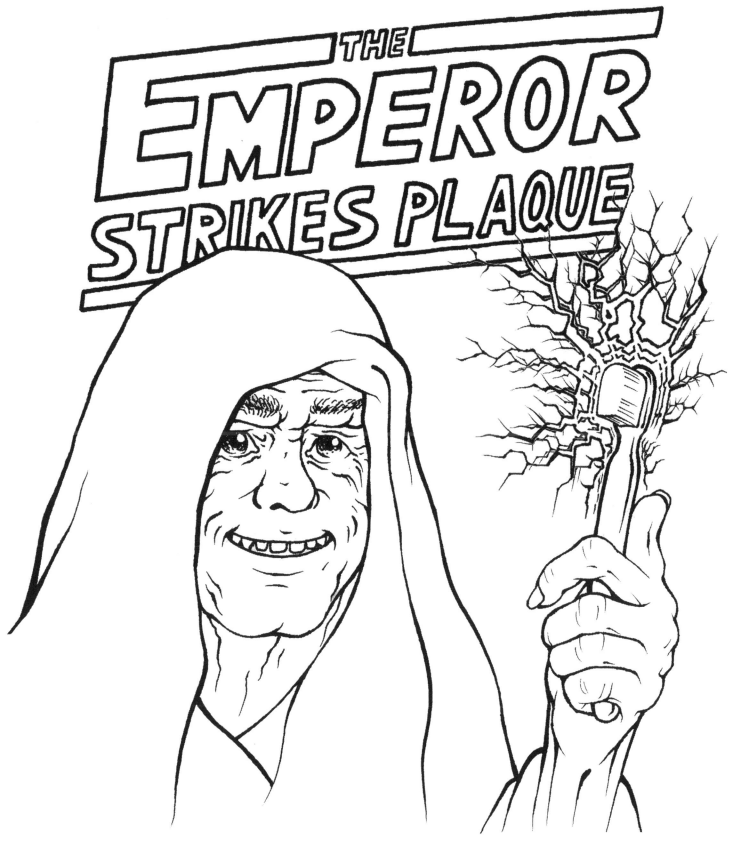

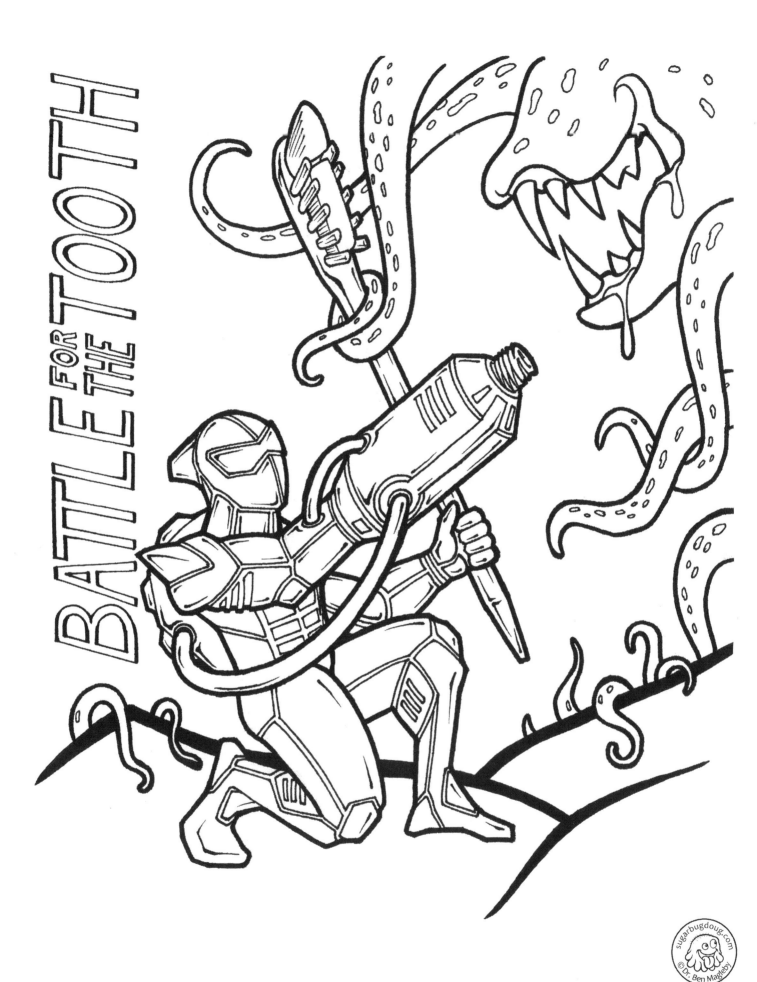

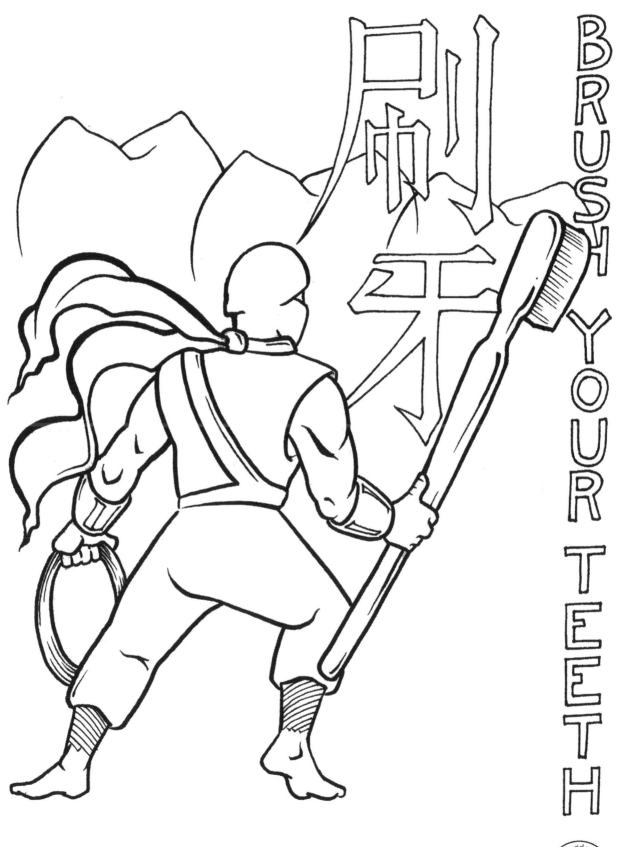

Dental Signs

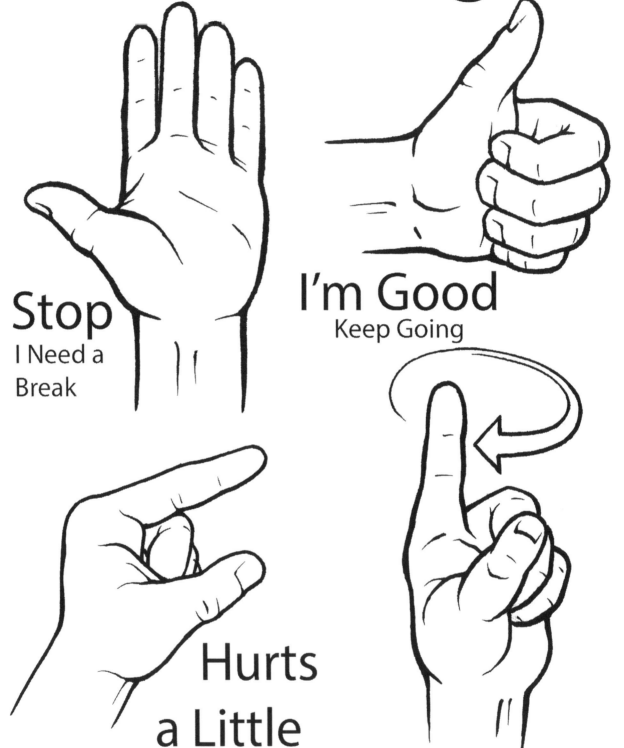

Stop
I Need a
Break

I'm Good
Keep Going

**Hurts
a Little**

Suction
Please Rinse My Mouth

lächeln sonreír

ابتسامة χαμόγελο

улыбка 微

হাসি

glimlach 笑

미소

スマイル

smile

רויח

 មញ្ញឹម mino'aka

ngiti sorridere

sorrir sourire

sugarbugdoug.com
©Dr. Ben Magleby

Crossword

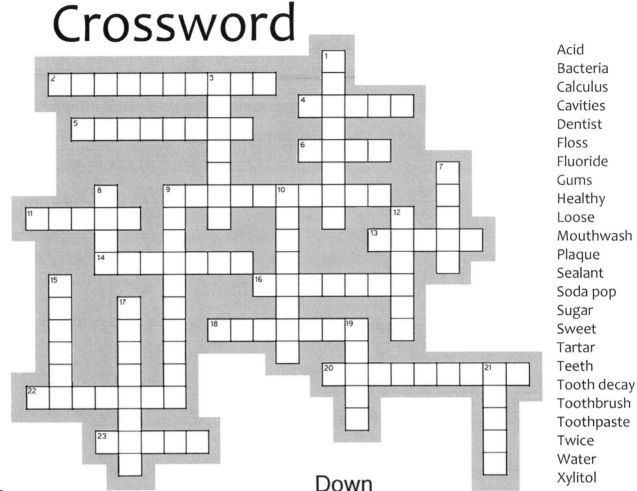

Acid
Bacteria
Calculus
Cavities
Dentist
Floss
Fluoride
Gums
Healthy
Loose
Mouthwash
Plaque
Sealant
Soda pop
Sugar
Sweet
Tartar
Teeth
Tooth decay
Toothbrush
Toothpaste
Twice
Water
Xylitol

Across

- Every day you should brush with _2_ and
  then _4_ your teeth.
- Toothpaste has _5_ in it to make your teeth strong.
- The "skin" around your teeth is called _6_ .
- You should brush with a _9_ at least _11_ a day.
- Rinsing with _13_ after meals helps prevent cavities.
- A _14_ can put a _16_ on your teeth to prevent cavities.
- Sugarless gum has _18_ in it, to stop bacteria
  from causing cavities.
- Rinsing with _20_ that has fluoride in it is
  another way to have _22_ _23_ .

Down

- When plaque stays in your mouth for a long time,
  it turns into _1_ .
- A drink that is filled with sugar as well as acid is _3_ .
- The bacteria in your mouth love to eat _7_ foods.
- When _8_ stays on your teeth for a long time
  it can cause _9_ .
- The germs in your mouth that cause cavities,
  plaque and calculus are _10_ .
  - When _15_ stays in your mouth for a long time,
    it turns into _12_ .
  - The rotten holes in your teeth called _17_
    are caused by bacteria that
    love to eat _21_ .
  - If you don't keep your teeth clean,
    then they can become _19_ , and fall out.

S	B	E	N	A	V	O	I	D	T	O	O	M	U	C	H	S	U	G	A	R	C
U	N	W	A	Z	E	V	K	F	C	J	Z	P	E	R	G	U	S	V	J	W	O
G	R	A	G	P	G	E	T	E	N	O	U	G	H	S	L	E	E	P	O	I	M
A	R	S	C	K	E	B	R	T	M	P	I	A	Q	B	G	X	T	A	R	E	P
R	B	H	T	K	T	Y	X	R	Z	Q	D	S	W	P	P	E	K	C	U	R	L
B	A	Y	W	P	A	J	E	A	T	F	R	E	S	H	F	R	U	I	T	V	E
U	L	O	V	E	B	L	X	N	K	Q	O	Y	U	I	L	C	O	D	O	N	X
G	A	U	T	K	L	P	L	A	Q	U	E	H	G	F	U	I	V	J	O	E	O
S	I	R	P	U	E	T	K	D	R	V	F	S	A	E	O	S	A	O	T	Q	R
T	O	H	I	E	S	E	A	C	A	N	D	Y	R	B	R	E	C	D	H	N	S
A	F	A	U	X	D	H	X	R	D	Y	C	V	H	N	I	N	X	O	P	V	I
H	L	N	J	P	M	Y	J	T	A	V	A	Y	F	C	D	Q	B	U	A	C	M
S	O	D	A	P	O	P	X	O	C	Y	V	N	E	V	E	N	Y	X	S	Y	P
X	S	S	E	F	U	K	J	O	F	Z	I	Y	D	E	N	T	I	S	T	H	L
W	S	W	F	S	T	B	X	T	K	A	T	D	B	G	Z	F	Z	N	E	S	E
H	E	A	L	T	H	Y	N	H	T	M	Y	J	H	J	E	G	C	O	H	P	C
B	J	H	O	R	W	X	J	B	Y	W	V	R	T	E	E	T	H	I	C	E	A
X	C	T	S	B	A	D	B	R	E	A	T	H	Z	Y	C	H	D	C	S	W	R
Y	S	M	S	Q	S	W	K	U	B	D	R	I	N	K	W	A	T	E	R	Q	B
F	M	T	P	R	H	K	M	S	N	S	N	Z	A	C	Y	N	M	D	C	R	O
G	I	Y	I	U	P	O	Q	H	Y	G	I	E	N	I	S	T	Q	W	E	A	H
J	L	K	C	O	O	K	I	E	R	N	W	E	B	R	D	A	B	C	L	T	Y
I	E	S	K	A	L	U	L	D	M	B	Z	M	W	N	C	R	D	Y	A	X	D
Q	P	Z	Q	G	U	M	K	V	C	S	E	A	L	A	N	T	R	I	U	T	R
L	Z	D	F	Z	K	G	H	J	B	V	K	R	Q	Z	B	A	F	C	G	V	A
C	B	R	U	S	H	T	W	I	C	E	A	D	A	Y	N	R	V	N	H	B	T
D	V	C	D	X	Q	Z	K	F	N	Q	C	N	B	R	F	D	Q	M	B	C	E
B	L	D	E	N	T	U	R	E	C	B	A	Q	K	C	A	L	C	U	L	U	S

Acid
Avoid too much sugar
Bad breath
Brush twice a day
Calculus
Candy
Cavity
Complex or simple
    carbohydrates
Cookie
Dentist
Denture
Drink water
Eat fresh fruit
Exercise
Floss
Floss pick
Fluoride
Get enough sleep
Gum
Healthy
Hygienist
Laugh
Mouthwash
Plaque
Sealant
Smile
Soda pop
Smack all day and
    get decay
Sugar
Sugarbugs
Tartar
Teeth
Toothbrush
Toothpaste
Vegetables
Wash your hands

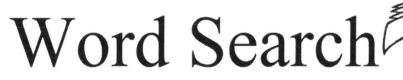

Word Search

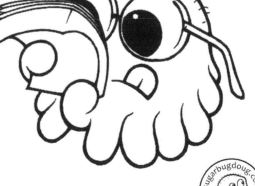

sugarbugdoug.com
© Dr. Ben Magleby

Tooth Erruption Chart

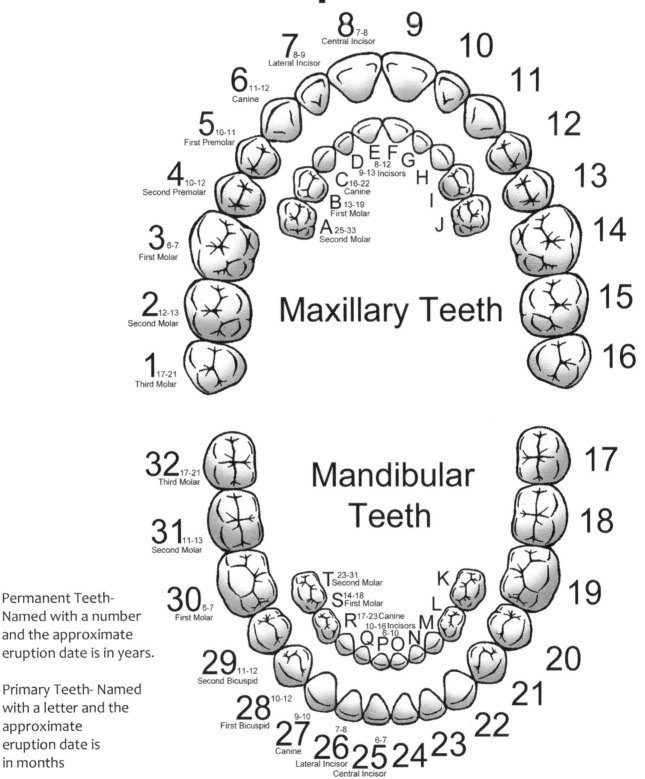

7 8-9 — Lateral Incisor
8 7-8 — Central Incisor
9
10
11
12
13
14
15
16

6 11-12 — Canine
5 10-11 — First Premolar
4 10-12 — Second Premolar
3 6-7 — First Molar
2 12-13 — Second Molar
1 17-21 — Third Molar

D
E
F
G — 8-12 9-13 Incisors
C 16-22 — Canine
B 13-19 — First Molar
A 25-33 — Second Molar
H
I
J

Maxillary Teeth

32 17-21 — Third Molar
31 11-13 — Second Molar
30 6-7 — First Molar
29 11-12 — Second Bicuspid
28 10-12 — First Bicuspid
27 9-10 — Canine
26 7-8 — Lateral Incisor
25 6-7 — Central Incisor
24
23
22
21
20
19
18
17

Mandibular Teeth

T 23-31 Second Molar
S 14-18 First Molar
R 17-23 Canine
10-16 Incisors
6-10
Q P O N
M
L
K

Permanent Teeth- Named with a number and the approximate eruption date is in years.

Primary Teeth- Named with a letter and the approximate eruption date is in months

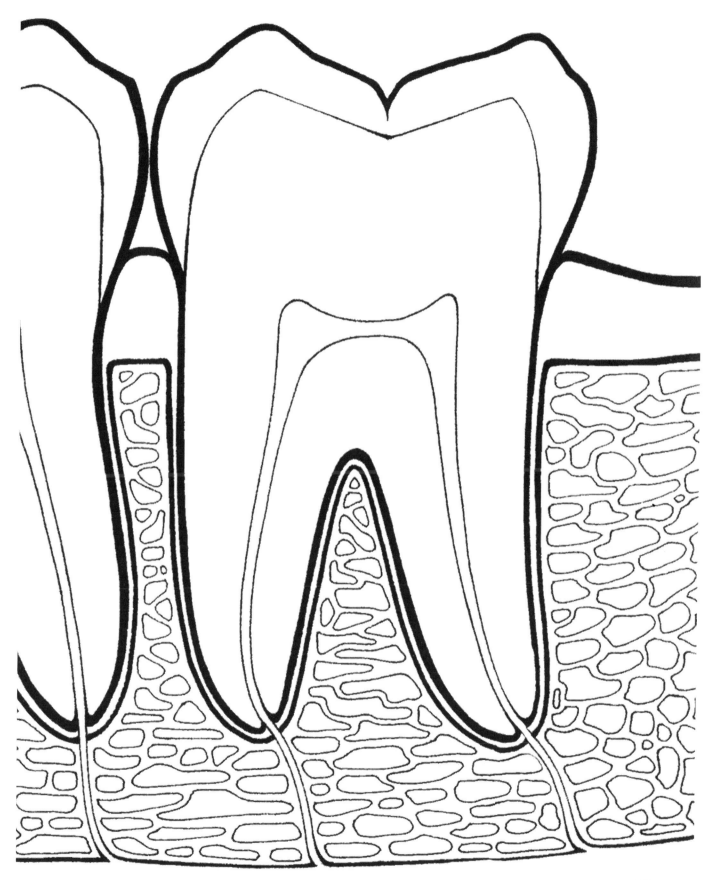

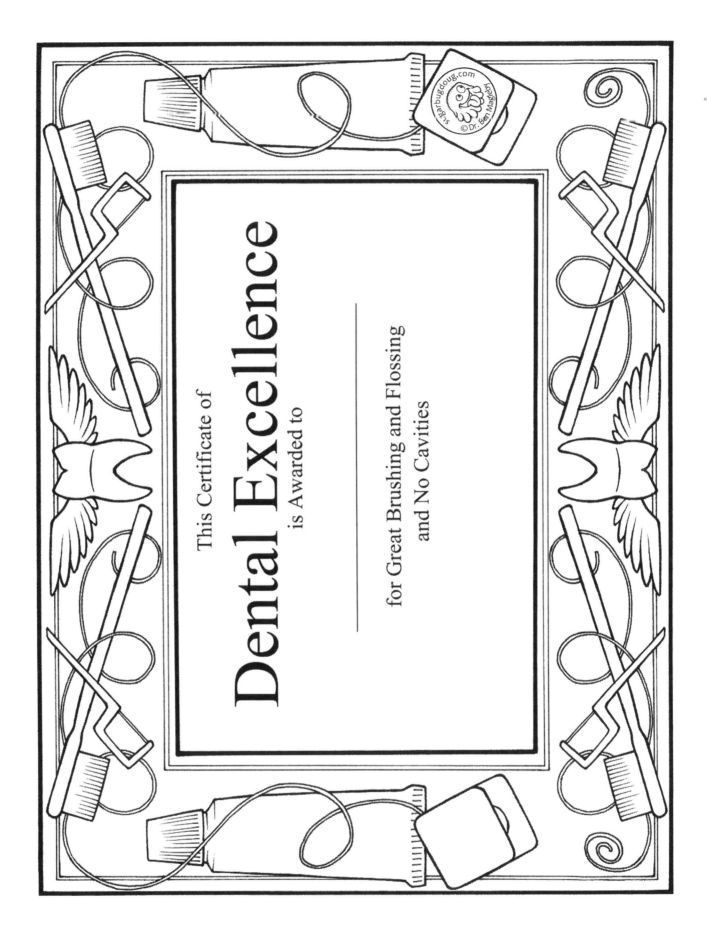

This Certificate of

Dental Excellence

is Awarded to

for Great Brushing and Flossing
and No Cavities

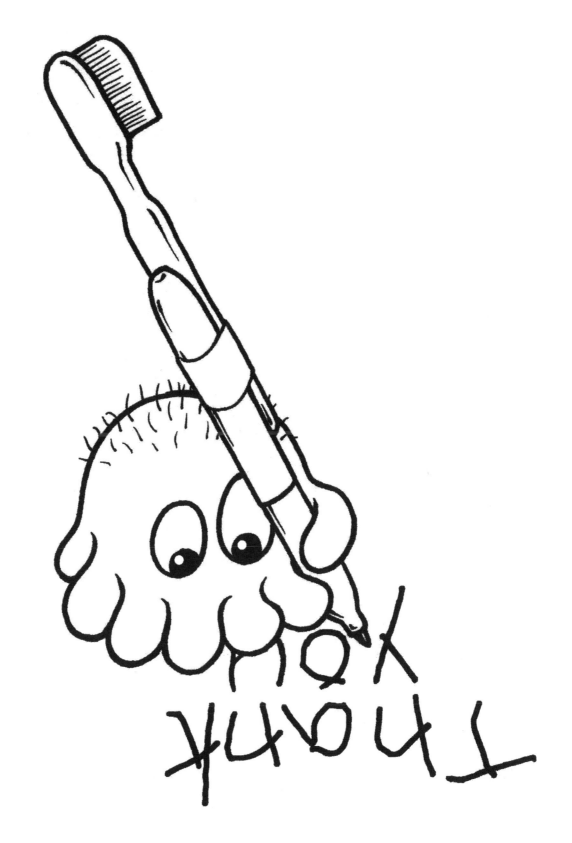

Key

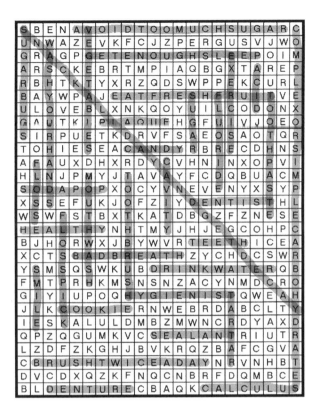

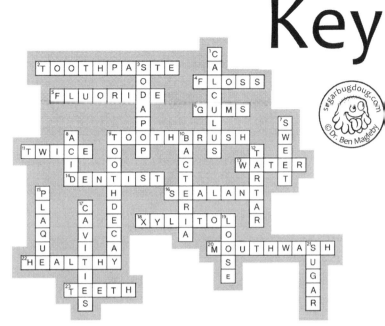

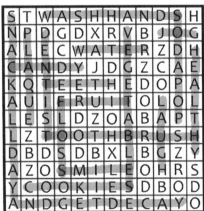

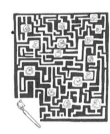

Maze: There are many right ways to finish the maze. The only goal is to get all of the sugarbugs. Like brushing for real, you need to clean all parts of all of your teeth.

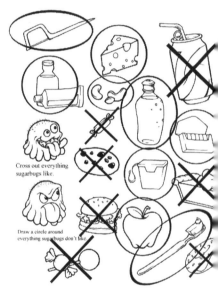

Cross out everything sugarbugs like.

Draw a circle around everything sugarbugs don't like.

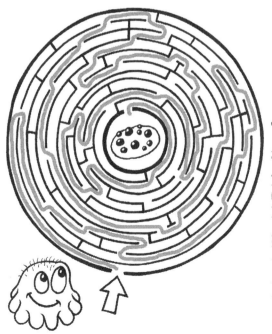

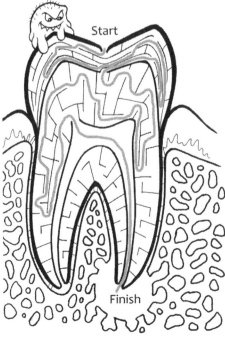

Start

Finish

Dot-to-Dot

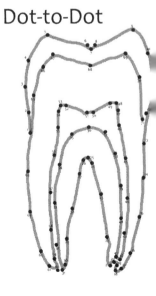

Made in the USA
Coppell, TX
07 January 2020